FACIAL FITNESS

FACIAL FITNESS

DAILY EXERCISES & MASSAGE TECHNIQUES FOR A HEALTHIER, YOUNGER LOOKING YOU

PATRICIA GOROWAY
Foreword by Dr. Richard H. Keller, DDS, MPS

BARNES & NOBLE
NEW YORK

Interior Design: Leah Lococo, Ltd.
Cover and Interior Illustrations: Monica Gurevich
Page 20: © Jon Feingersh/zefa/Corbis; Page 21L: © Nad Images/Getty;
Page 21R: © Daly & Newton/Getty;
Pages 43–45: © S. Karger AG, Basel, Switzerland

2006 Barnes & Noble

Library of Congress Cataloging-in-Publication Data

Goroway, Patricia.
Facial fitness : daily exercise and massage techniques for a healthier, younger looking you / Patricia Goroway.
p. cm.
ISBN-13: 978-0-7607-8094-7 (alk. paper)   ISBN-10: 0-7607-8094-3 (alk. paper)
1. Facial exercises. 2. Face—Massage. 3. Beauty, Personal. I. Title.
RA778b.G67 2006   646.7'2—dc22   2006015945

Printed and bound in China by Millenium International, Ltd.

3   5   7   9   10   8   6   4   2

DEDICATION

This book is dedicated to my father, Ronald James Connolly, 1935–2006.

ACKNOWLEDGMENTS

I would like to thank the many friends, colleagues, editors, and medical professionals who have assisted me in writing this book, including:

Nathaniel Marunas, Betsy Beier, and Devorah Klein at Barnes & Noble for their skill and support, and for making this project a reality.

Dr. Richard Keller for introducing me to the possibilities of facial exercising.

My father, Ronald Connolly for his love, knowledge, and support, and for making me aware of the questionable ingredients used in skin care products.

Erik, Grace, and Joanna for their friendship, love, and encouragement through a difficult time.

David, for sharing his brilliant ideas and insights. And to my sons, Travis and Hunter, for their love, and for making me so proud.

All who contributed to this work with their personal and professional knowledge. Their input is greatly appreciated.

CONTENTS

FOREWORD

As A BIOLOGICAL dentist who focuses on head and neck pain and temporomandibular joint (TMJ) dysfunction, nothing is more gratifying than patients who ultimately become pain-free, and who embrace healthy habits that ensure they remain pain-free. I have found that recommending exercises as prescribed in Patricia Goroway's *Facial Fitness* is necessary to support this healing process. Not only do Ms. Goroway's detailed exercises and regimens promote natural healing and muscle tonus, they result in healthier skin and a tighter face, giving readers a more youthful appearance.

Whether you have sought surgical or non-surgical solutions for maintaining the appearance of your early years, this book's holistic, noninvasive approach will help rejuvenate your face and neck. Readers will find that the detailed and clear instructions easily facilitate a continued commitment to vibrant, glowing, and—most importantly—well-toned skin. I know: I have been practicing the exercises and massage techniques since I received the manuscript!

In addition to exercises, massage techniques, and a regimen to support the muscles of the face and neck, *Facial Fitness* provides crucial information about utilizing well-chosen, natural skin products that will achieve the best results for your skin. (All beauty products are not alike!) It will also introduce you to high standards of integrating good lifestyle choices such as drinking plenty of clean, non-chemically tainted water; consuming vitamins, minerals, and healthful food; and aerobically exercising all your muscle groups; which will promote the body's own capabilities to heal, rejuvenate, and obtain optimal health.

Now that *Facial Fitness* is available, I intend to recommend it to my temporomandibular dysfunction patients, who I am sure will benefit immensely from the step-by-step explanations for the exercises and massages. During my last forty years of practicing dentistry, I have found that people with good physical and mental health radiate youthfulness and vitality. So whether you are using the exercises and massage techniques for rehabilitation, simple toning to decrease wrinkles, or to maintain surgical alterations, *Facial Fitness* is sure to be very useful to your physical and emotional health.

—Dr. Richard H. Keller, DDS, MPS

INTRODUCTION

Y EARS AGO, after what was to be
a life-changing automobile accident, I discovered the amazing effects that exercising
the muscles of the face and neck had on
the injuries I sustained during that accident.
The experience was life-changing because it
left me with a newfound recognition that
it is often possible to find alternatives to the
generally prescribed course of treatment.
I suffered a debilitating injury involving my
neck and my temporomandibular joint, or
TMJ. I had incredibly sharp pain that ran
across my face. My bottom jaw was left
misaligned and glided to one side when
I opened my mouth. It popped and cracked

so loudly whenever I tried to eat solid
food that the sound was audible to others
around me.

A surgical specialist advised me that
surgery was the only way to minimize
my pain and restore normal form and
function to my face. The proposed procedure required incisions to be made on
both sides of my face (possibly leaving
scars) in an attempt to tighten the muscles
and ligaments and hopefully relieve the
pain and correct the misalignment. There
was no guarantee this procedure would
work, and my mouth would be wired
shut, which meant that I would be on a
strictly liquid diet for a sustained period
of time.

Thankfully, I sought a second opinion
and was directed to a physician specializing
in facial and cranial rehabilitation. His

approach included treating the injuries with a series of strengthening exercises to help eliminate the pain and correct the misalignment naturally. As clumsy and difficult as they were to perform, the exercises really worked. Within a month the pain was gone. But what happened next was truly amazing: not only were the muscles that had been directly affected by the injury toned, tightened, and pain free, but so were the surrounding muscles.

I have always been acutely aware of the importance of good skin-care. When I was a child, my father was in the cosmetics and skin-care industry and had access to the latest research and developments in the field. From an early age, he taught me the importance of good skin-care and how to be aware of the ingredients that cosmetic products contain.

As an adult, I became even more interested in the field and paid close attention to the latest information and so-called "breakthrough" skin-care and cosmetic products and procedures. When I visited my dermatologist for various conditions, I made a point of asking her opinion about the latest products and options. The options sounded promising, but somewhat limited. After all, just applying moisturizer to our bodies does not produce toned muscles. I was sure there was more that people could do to improve their skin.

After my accident, I began to conduct even more detailed research about the face, and in particular, its muscles, by consulting medical specialists, reading medical journals, and learning everything I could about how and why these muscles respond so well to exercise. I soon discovered that the muscles of the face and neck are all con-nected in a striated, quilt-like structure that lies just below the surface of the skin. Interwoven by fibers, the muscles are attached to each other, to the bone, and to the skin. They work synergistically to help you do everything from smiling and frowning to chewing, whistling, breathing, and even swallowing. Every expression you make, as well as every emotion and reaction you experience, is displayed on your face because of the connection of these muscles to specific cranial nerves whose nuclei lay within the brain stem. The science is complicated, but here's the bottom line: scientists believe that the muscles of the face and neck are unique because of their involuntary link to your emotional processes. They also believe that no other animal has evolved

as complex a set of facial muscles as humans have.

Scientists believe that the muscles of the face and neck are unique because of their involuntary link to your emotional processes.

I was fascinated by the information I discovered and the results I achieved by doing the facial exercises recommended to me by my doctor. I decided that I wanted to develop a series of exercises that would target all the muscles of the face and neck and create a complete facial exercise program. So, I continued my research. I studied anatomy and asked lots of questions to anyone I came across in the medical, health, or beauty industry. The common theme I came across again and again was that exercising the muscles of the face and neck is extremely beneficial to laying the groundwork for a youthful complexion.

So, how does it work? Through my research, I learned that the supply of blood to a contracting muscle is ten times greater than it is to a muscle at rest. This fresh blood supply delivers vital oxygen and nutrients to the skin and revitalizes the tissues. It is an all too common practice for people, especially women, to attempt to tighten the skin over a slack underlying structure through the use of plastic surgery,

only to have the inevitable effects of gravity cause the face to appear droopy once again.

With that in mind, I began to adapt the basic maneuvers I had learned during my rehabilitation into a series of facial exercises that would work many of the fifty-seven muscles of the face and neck. The results were phenomenal. Not only were my muscles becoming toned and tightened, but fine lines and wrinkles began to fill in, erasing the signs of aging. And that was only the beginning. I then developed a series of facial massage techniques that were specifically designed to accompany and enhance the facial exercise program. After years of research and fine-tuning, the Facial Fitness program was born.

Many people resort to cosmetic procedures to improve their appearance. However, as I myself found out, these procedures are temporary and can be quite costly, especially when you have to keep repeating them every few months to maintain the desired effects. So, why not try exercising first? You will see the change in your appearance almost immediately, and in time you will be able to sculpt your face as you would your body, through strength training, to achieve a more youthful, radiant look.

I've never been afraid to try new things, but I have usually preferred a natural approach to improving my health and appearance whenever possible. I believe in seeking out alternative methods for improving one's health and appearance without the use of surgery. Developing the Facial Fitness program was simply a logical progression for me to rehabilitate, improve, and maintain a healthy, youthful complexion.

Because the muscles of the face and neck are smaller than most other muscles in the body, they respond very quickly to exercise. As a result, my facial exercise regimen, in conjunction with the facial massage techniques I've incorporated into the program, will erase years of aging in just weeks. And, with regular practice, you will maintain that youthful, healthy look for years to come.

My goal is to offer an alternative to costly and potentially risky procedures (after all, every surgery carries risks, no matter how well established the procedure is) and to help you cultivate a more natural-looking beauty by simply exercising your way to a more youthful complexion. However, if you choose to have surgery, these exercises do not interfere with or contradict any previous facial surgery or cosmetic treatment. As a matter of fact, the program works very well to help maintain the results you may achieve after such procedures.

❦ ❦ ❦

. . . you will be able to sculpt your face as you would your body, through strength training, to achieve a more youthful, radiant look.

❦ ❦ ❦

Lawrence Birnbaum, M.D., a Beverly Hills plastic surgeon says, "Exercises are extremely beneficial to both pre– and post–operative cosmetic surgery patients.

Exercises can also help anyone lift sagging facial skin via building up the fifty-seven facial muscles."

I wrote this book to share what I have learned: how and why to perform facial exercises and massage techniques. I also wanted to offer a comprehensive guide to healthy approaches to skin-care based on the research and information I have gathered. My hope is that once you have this information in hand, you will begin to make healthier choices, because let's face it—everyone wants to look younger. You just need to know how to achieve that goal without putting yourself at risk. If you can do something that immediately improves your looks while also improving your overall health, then you will truly have something to smile about.

PART ONE

CHAPTER 1

HOW AND WHY THE SKIN AGES

RESEARCH shows that there are two types of aging. Aging caused by the genes you are born with is called intrinsic (internal or chronological) aging, and aging caused by external factors, such as the environment, is referred to as extrinsic aging. Intrinsic aging is a natural process that involves, among other things, the shortening of the life span of your cells. By the time you are an adult, the life span of your cells is less than half of what it was when you were a child. For example, it takes you longer to heal from cuts and scrapes, you begin to bruise more easily, your circulation decreases, and toxins are eliminated at a slower rate. This is the normal aging process, and there's not much we can do to stop it. The factors affecting extrinsic aging, however, can be controlled, so it is these that we will focus on in this chapter.

In your **twenties,** your skin appears firm and virtually wrinkle free. However, within the skin, the production of both collagen and elastin—the substances that enable skin to bounce back from sun exposure, wounds, acne, and the like—slows down. This process is accelerated by repeated exposure to the sun's harmful ultraviolet (UV) rays.

This, along with a slight decrease in the ability of dead skin cells to shed, begins the signs of intrinsic aging. Failing to properly protect your skin from the sun's damaging rays at this age (as many people do), and other unhealthy lifestyle choices often made by the young and uninitiated, causes long-term damage and exacerbates the visible signs of aging. Although the signs might not become noticeable until you are well into your thirties, the inevitable process of aging has begun.

In your **thirties,** lines begin to form around the eyes, called crow's-feet, between the brows, called glabellar lines, and on the forehead, called transverse lines. Collagen and elastin production continues to slow down, and the skin becomes puffier, especially around the eye area. How you protect, treat, nourish, and strengthen your skin at this age can mean a great deal when it comes to your long-term health and beauty. As you grow older, it will make the difference between looking younger than you are, or, unfortunately, looking much older.

In your **forties,** you can expect to see an even greater loss of elasticity in the skin. The face also begins to lose volume as the skin's fat and collagen begins to diminish. The skin becomes more transparent, the corners of the mouth start to turn down, and age spots may appear or darken. The skin may also become drier due to decreased levels of estrogen.

In your **fifties,** gravity really starts to have an impact. It causes the tip of the nose to droop, the ears to elongate, the eyelids to fall, and the jowls to become more pronounced.

In your **sixties and beyond,** the impact of gravity that you began to see in your fifties becomes even more pronounced. In addition, your face can appear to be puffy and tired all day. Inflammation and fluid build-up are more prevalent at this point, as are fatty deposits under the eyes and chin.

Intrinsic aging is inevitable, however there are ways to help slow the effects of this natural process. One of the most important ways to decelerate the aging clock is to make sure you are nourishing your body properly. Good nutrition is essential, but you have to eat what is right for you. Many people suffer from food intolerances and allergies and do not even know it. Oftentimes, unbeknownst to you, the food you most enjoy may be causing digestive problems and headaches, and sapping your energy. You may not see the correlation between what you're eating and how you feel afterwards. If you suffer from any of these symptoms, it's not a bad idea to consult your physician, as well as a nutritionist, and adopt a diet plan that's right for your body.

In addition to proper nutrition, it is essential to get plenty of sleep and drink lots of water, preferably with lemon. As you may know, lemon contains lots of vitamin C and helps reduce inflammation. Try to minimize stress through exercise and massage, and of course, do not smoke!

❧ ❧ ❧

One of the most important ways to decelerate the aging clock is to make sure you are nourishing your body properly.

❧ ❧ ❧

Extrinsic aging is responsible for most of the visible signs of prematurely aged skin. One example of this type of aging is prolonged exposure to the sun's harmful UV rays, which is called photoaging. Although it may seem as if these signs appear out of nowhere (often in the form of wrinkles), they have actually been building up under the skin's surface for years. With repeated exposure to the sun, the skin loses the ability to repair itself; thus the damage accumulates. Most skin cancer occurs in prematurely aged skin. Increasing numbers of cases of melanoma (skin cancer) have been well documented in the last few years, perhaps due to the depletion of the ozone. But one thing is for sure: permanent skin damage and disease occurs because of accumulated destruction within the skin from previous years of prolonged sun exposure. That is why it is essential for you take steps now to protect not only yourself but your children as well from further damage that could lead to skin cancer. By educating your children and applying sunscreen to their skin whenever they are exposed to sunlight for extended amounts of time, you can help protect them from the harmful effects of the sun's burning rays. After just a few instances of being sunburned as a child, a person is

"I have been using the Facial Fitness exercises for about a month and a half, and I can see a big difference in my skin. My jawline has tightened quite a bit, the wrinkles on my forehead are almost gone, and my brow area has lifted a little. I am quite happy with the program."

—RITA MOLFETAS

already at an increased risk of developing skin cancer later in life.

The scientific details of how and why the sun damages your skin are very technical, but suffice it to say that it's essential to protect your skin as much as possible if you want to avoid skin cancer and premature aging. A few ways to ensure that you are being protected from the sun's harmful rays is to wear protective clothing, including a hat and sunglasses, and use sunscreen on a daily basis—no matter what time of year or in what climate. Many excellent skin-care lines now contain a broad-spectrum sunscreen with an SPF (sun protection factor) of fifteen or higher in their day-creams, so it is very simple to protect your skin as you moisturize. Make sure that the products you apply contain both UVA and UVB protection, and apply a moisturizer with sunblock liberally,

letting it dry completely before applying your makeup or putting on clothing.

e❦ e❦ e❦

After just a few instances of being sunburned as a child, a person is already at an increased risk of developing skin cancer later in life.

e❦ e❦ e❦

In addition to the sun, the skin has many more enemies. Among them are smoking, excess alcohol consumption, crash dieting, dehydration, exposure to chemicals contained in some cosmetics and skin-care products, pollution, and stress, just to name a few. Each of these, in its own sinister way, damages the skin. Some cause deterioration of collagen and elastin, others may interfere with the rate at which new cells turn over. This kind of damage dramatically affects the skin's tone and outer appearance. Because of this, fine lines, wrinkles, and skin discoloration begin to occur, and skin begins to age prematurely.

It is essential to minimize exposure to those sources of skin damage mentioned above by taking preventative steps to ensure as little damage to the skin as possible. No one wants to accelerate the aging process, but unfortunately an unhealthy lifestyle does just that.

As you learn to avoid these potentially harmful factors and begin a healthy routine of skin-care, it is vital to add a facial exercise and massage program to your daily

"This is the greatest thing I've done for my appearance yet. The results I've seen after just a few weeks are remarkably noticeable, and it was so easy. I highly recommend it to anyone looking for a safe, effective alternative to surgery."

—LINDA CONNOLLY

regimen so that you don't neglect the muscles of the face and neck. Simply moving your face by making various expressions or eating does not mean all the muscles are being worked and strengthened effectively. Consistently exercising and massaging the facial muscles properly will ensure a more youthful and toned appearance for years to come.

৬❀ ৬❀ ৬❀

Exercise and massage are intrinsic parts of a healthy lifestyle, so why not have your face benefit as well?

৬❀ ৬❀ ৬❀

Through exercise and massage, the muscles become toned and circulation increases, thus allowing the waste products and toxins trapped within the skin's layers to be eliminated more efficiently. Exercise also helps stimulate the skin, giving it a youthful glow. The massage program alone provides both immediate and long-term benefits, not the least of which is a reduction in stress, but when used in conjunction with the facial exercises, a healthy, firm foundation is formed on which to build and maintain youthful-looking skin.

By following the Facial Fitness program and adopting a proactive skin-care regimen, you will be able to actually reverse many of the visible signs of aging by protecting, strengthening, and toning the facial muscles. Your cheeks will seem less hollow, the corners of your mouth will be lifted, your eyes will widen, your neck will become smoother, and your jowls will begin to lift.

As you know, a healthy lifestyle, good nutrition, and plenty of rest will greatly improve your overall health. Exercise and massage are intrinsic parts of a healthy lifestyle, so why not have your face benefit as well? So much about the way you feel is projected on your face. When someone is truly healthy in mind and body you can see it immediately. She or he exudes confidence and well-being, which is very attractive to others. It's quite simple—when you look good, you feel good. The Facial Fitness program is an all-natural way to promote a healthy, youthful appearance. Follow the program carefully, and in no time you will begin to see amazing results right before your eyes. Your facial features will become more defined, and you will be able to sculpt your face as you would your body, through the use of specific exercises designed to enhance your own natural beauty.

"I can't believe the results I experienced after just two weeks of using the Facial Fitness system. My jawline is tighter and the lines around my eyes have just about vanished. It's incredible!"

—GRACE SURDIS

CHAPTER 2

THE BENEFITS OF FACIAL EXERCISE

FACIAL EXERCISE AND MASSAGE have many benefits. Not only will they tone and tighten the muscles of the face and neck, but they will instantly rejuvenate tired looking skin by increasing the blood flow and circulation, revitalizing the skin's surface with a flushed, healthy glow. The exercises are great to do as a quick pick-me-up whenever you want to look rested and refreshed, and you will see the long-term benefits of reduced wrinkles and an overall younger look in no time.

Here is what you will achieve by following the Facial Fitness program:

- A youthful, healthy appearance

- The appearance of a longer neck through proper posture

- An evenly balanced head by strengthening the neck muscles

- A clear, radiant complexion by helping to release toxins from the skin and increase circulation

- A relaxed forehead by training the muscles to be at ease

- Uplifted eyes by strengthening the muscles above the eyes

- Raised eyebrows through toning the muscles above the brow

- Firmer cheeks by strengthening the facial and jaw muscles

- Upturned corners of the mouth by toning the nasal-labial muscles

- Fuller, smoother lips by toning and relaxing the muscles around the mouth

- A well-shaped nose by toning the nasal muscles and thinning the appearance of the nose

- A well-shaped jawline by lifting the muscles of the face and neck

- Increased awareness of your facial expressions through a conscious effort to visualize each and every muscle as it is being trained and strengthened

- Better control of your facial expressions as you become aware of the facial muscles and how they react when a particular emotion is portrayed

🌀 Alleviated symptoms of TMJ disorder by strengthening the muscles and ligaments and encouraging increased circulation to the affected area

🌀 Alleviated symptoms of Bell's palsy by strengthening the affected muscles or group of muscles and learning to relax them

Not only does the Facial Fitness program help maintain a youthful appearance, but it can relieve painful facial conditions. For years, specialized physical therapists and physicians have been prescribing facial exercises as part of a rehabilitation regimen for the treatment of conditions such as TMJ disorder and Bell's palsy. Facial resistance training is now being offered at many rehabilitation facilities to address these conditions. Studies showing their effectiveness are readily available online.

Bell's palsy is a sudden and debilitating condition that is a type of paralysis or weakness of the muscles in the face, thought to be due to inflammation of the seventh cranial nerve, also known as the facial nerve. Gaye Cronin, OTD, OTR, the director of the Neuromuscular Facial Retraining Program at the Atlanta Ear Clinic, says, "Loss of facial function can affect a person's quality of life, self-esteem, oral motor controls, and eyelid function. Other problems can develop as well, such as abnormal movement patterns, abnormal tone, eye irritations, and taste or chewing problems." Bell's palsy can be effectively treated by performing targeted facial exercises. Of course, you should always consult your doctor before performing any exercise regimen, especially one designed to relieve a particular condition. Todd Henkelmann, PT, MS, of the University of Pittsburgh Medical Center Facial Nerve Center, says that those suffering from acute cases of Bell's palsy should not perform exercises during the first few weeks of the syndrome, due to flaccidity of the affected side.

Through the use of facial neuromuscular training, strength and stability can be restored to the affected area of the face. Authorities on Bell's palsy recommend that patients familiarize themselves with the muscles of the face and neck to help isolate the muscle action, and they also suggest performing the exercises in front of a mirror to ensure that they are being done properly and effectively. Additionally, many authorities recommend massage as part of the routine in all stages of recovery.

Gaye Cronin adds that, "Neuromuscular facial retraining programs have proven to be successful in the recovery of facial function. Facial exercises for specific, isolated movements are included in these programs." The following are examples of functional facial exercises created by Cronin to help alleviate symptoms of Bell's palsy. If you suffer from Bell's palsy, practice these exercises once a day, in addition to my recommended exercises later in the book.

❀ ❀ ❀

When rehabilitation is the goal, remember to work the muscles gently as you progress though your routine and do not overwork any one area.

❀ ❀ ❀

- **To increase eyelid closure:** Hold a target approximately 25 degrees below eye level. Keep your eyes on the target and slowly lower your eyelids. Try not to allow your eyeballs to roll up or out. Try to keep the target in focus until the lids completely close.

- **To increase lip closure:** Face a mirror and press your lips together. Hold for 5 counts, then move your lips into a pucker position and hold for 5 counts. Try to keep your lips centered and do not allow them to pull toward the stronger side.

- **To decrease synkinesis (abnormal movement patterns):** Face a mirror and make small puckers with your mouth. As soon as you see or feel your eyelid muscles pull or squint, stop the mouth movement. Make a conscious effort to isolate the mouth movements from the eye movements.

When rehabilitation is the goal, remember to work the muscles gently as you progress though your routine, and do not overwork any one area. Symmetry and balance, as well as regained movement, are the goals when exercising for medical reasons, so do not overdo it. Exercise in short sessions and stop when you begin to feel fatigued. Exercises and massage techniques recommended specifically for the rehabilitation of Bell's palsy are discussed later in the book.

Temporomandibular joint disorder, or TMJ disorder, is another common condition affecting millions of people. This extremely painful disorder stems from an unwanted deviation of the jaw when the patient opens his or her mouth. TMJ disorder usually occurs when the teeth are misaligned or a person suffers an injury, such as a blow to the face, or an indirect trauma, such as whiplash, which causes a displacement of the cartilage where the jaw is attached to the skull. This displacement in turn causes a painful sense of pressure and stretching of the associated sensory nerves. Another condition known as bruxism, which is an abnormal grinding of the teeth, is also a leading cause of TMJ disorder. Bruxism is usually accompanied by a popping or clicking of the jaw, as well as sharp, sudden pain, which may radiate up and across the face.

Facial exercises are used to help re-educate the jaw to open correctly, thus alleviating many of these symptoms. According to Dr. Richard H. Keller, DDS,

of the American Academy of Biomechanical Trauma and Cranio-Facial Pain, "Facial exercises, especially for the muscles of mastication and those involving the tongue, are very effective in the realignment of the jaw and help to alleviate the pressure and pain associated with TMJ disorder. Approximately 85 percent of the patients using these exercises, often called neuromuscular reeducation, experience success. Others may need further treatment, such as injections known as neuraltherapy and/or the use of a splint to further alleviate pain and correct any misalignment."

The Facial Fitness program was originated with TMJ disorders in mind and has been proven effective in alleviating many of the symptoms associated with it when the exercises and massage techniques are performed on a consistent basis. You'll find specific exercises and massage techniques for the rehabilitation of TMJ disorder later in the book.

As with any exercise program, consistency is the key to success, so make the Facial Fitness program part of your everyday routine, whether your goal is rehabilitation or just simple toning. Before long you will begin to see and feel results.

CHAPTER 3

THE MUSCLES AND HOW THEY WORK

ON THE FOLLOWING PAGES are diagrams of the head, face, and neck muscles. As you will see, they form a complex and intricate system that works synergistically to provide form and function, as well as to express emotion. Like all our muscles, if they are left static, they begin to slacken over time, creating the appearance of tired, aged, unhealthy skin. For example, when your face is at rest while you are reading, sleeping, driving, watching television, working on the computer, or listening intently, it is generally motionless. Unless you are making some involuntary movements such as pursing your lips or squinting, the muscles on your face are, for the most part, not engaged.

❧ ❧ ❧

Once you become aware of the way you look when you are occupied with a specific task or deep in thought, you can begin to train your "facial posture."

❧ ❧ ❧

Have you ever unexpectedly caught a glimpse of yourself in a mirror? Were you surprised to see the expression you were making? Most of the time we are not aware of what we truly look like. Once you become aware of the way you look when you are occupied with a specific task or deep in thought, you can begin to train your "facial posture." Much like becoming aware of your body's posture and straightening up when you slouch, you should become aware of your facial posture and do the same. Incorporating a facial exercise routine into your everyday life is a terrific way to tone and tighten these muscles.

Actors are often taught to become acutely aware of their facial expressions and some are even trained to perform facial exercises to make themselves fully conscious of each expression they're making. Having command of these muscles helps actors convey to the audience the emotions they intend to project so that their characters are believable and convincing.

"I am a method actor in New York who has been using facial exercises for years without even knowing it. In the method I use, it is a process of complete body relaxation. The theory is that the more relaxed you are the easier it is to draw on a sense memory for whatever role you are playing. When I first started taking acting classes, my instructor showed us facial exercises to get in touch with the muscles in the face. When you are in tune with your muscles and aware of any stress you may be holding in these muscles, it becomes easier to relax them. The instructors informed us that one of the by-products of these exercises would be a more youthful appearance. Being an actor approaching forty years old, this can come in pretty handy. When one of my friends told me about the Facial Fitness program, I was very excited and had to check it out. The first time I watched the DVD, I was hooked. For years I have been struggling with the muscles in my forehead. I could never seem to relax them, which has given me wrinkles. Not only has the Facial Fitness program brought me more in tune with these muscles, but my wrinkles are starting to go away."

—GEORGE NETZ

Listed from top to bottom are the major muscles of the head, face, and neck and a brief description of their function. Diagrams of the muscles can be found on pages 43 to 45.

MUSCLES OF THE SCALP

The *galea aponeurotica* is a flat tendon that covers the top part of the cranium and connects the *frontalis* and the *occipitalis* muscles.

The *occipitalis* is a small muscle located at the back of the head. It is part of the muscle group that moves the scalp.

The *frontalis* is the muscle that covers the forehead. In conjunction with the *corrugator*, it is responsible for raising and lowering the scalp, forehead, eyebrows, and the top of the nose. Constantly raising and lowering the eyebrows through expression causes deep horizontal lines across the forehead. Toning

these muscles properly will help to smooth out these lines, and make you more aware of your facial expressions.

MUSCLES OF THE EYE

There are several muscles in the eye area. The *orbicularis oculi* is primarily responsible for the opening and closing of the eye, and the *procerus* is responsible for the movement of the skin between the eyebrows.

The *levator palpebrae,* the muscle found behind the *orbicularis oculi* in the upper eyelid, is also responsible for the opening and closing of the eye.

Strengthening these muscles will help to fight the gravitational pull on these delicate areas of the face. Squinting causes many of the lines and wrinkles that surround the eyes and betray your age. You can diminish the signs of aging caused by sun exposure by protecting your eyes from the sun by wearing sunblock and sunglasses.

MUSCLES OF THE NOSE

Yes, even the nose has muscles. Try flaring your nostrils and you will feel the anterior and posterior *dilatator* muscles working to increase the airflow through the nose.

The *nasalis,* which is located over the bridge of the nose, helps compress the nostrils, as does the *depressor septi.* Strengthening these muscles will help reshape the nose and prevent the tip from drooping.

MUSCLES OF THE MOUTH

The muscles responsible for opening and closing the mouth are known as the *orbicularis oris* and the *caninus.* These muscles completely surround the mouth and are connected to the nose, cheeks, lips, and chin.

The *mentalis* is located on the front of the chin. It raises and lowers the chin and lower lip. The *quadratus labii superioris* lies above the top lip and the *quadratus labii inferioris* lies below the lower lip.

MUSCLES OF MASTICATION

The muscles of mastication—including the *pterygoideus internus,* the *pterygoideus externus,* the *masseter,* the *temporalis,* and the *buccinator*—work together to give the jaw the ability to operate in all of its vital functions, such as opening and closing the mouth, chewing, grinding, yawning, and, of course, speaking. Toning these muscles helps alleviate the appearance of facial drooping and can relieve the painful symptoms of TMJ disorder.

MUSCLES OF THE NECK

Known as the *platysma* muscles, the muscles of the neck run from the corners of the mouth to the jaw, and down to the collarbone in the front of the neck on either side. They assist in the operation of the jaw and help with swallowing. As you age, these muscles start to separate, causing the appearance of cords running down either side of the neck, sometimes with loose skin in between. The *sternocleidomastoid* is primarily responsible for turning the head from side to side, and along with the *trapezesius* muscle, allows you to partially rotate the head, as well as move it up and down.

Now that you are familiar with these major muscles of the face and neck, you will be able to focus on them as you isolate a particular muscle or group of muscles and visualize them as you tone and strengthen them through the Facial Fitness program.

There's no time like the present, so let's get you started on your way to a more youthful, healthy, and dynamic appearance. Remember: repetition is essential to your success, so stick with it, and in no time you will begin to see results. This remarkable method of strengthening will give a natural lift to your face and neck—and take years off your appearance.

MUSCLES OF THE HEAD, FACE, AND NECK
(FRONTAL VIEW)

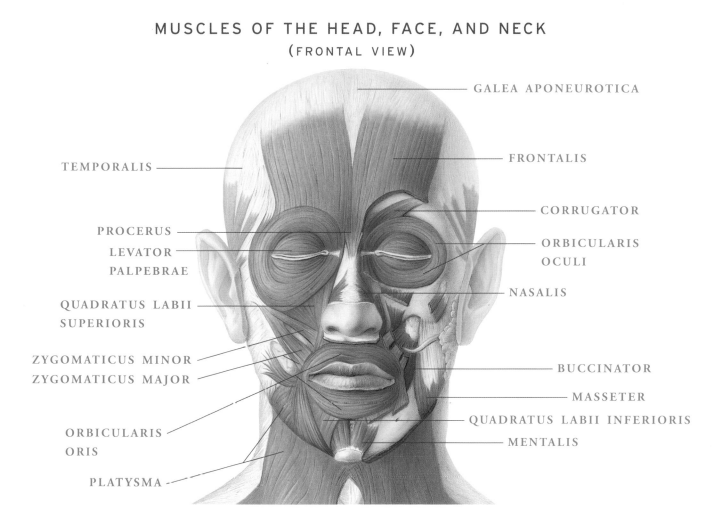

GALEA APONEUROTICA

FRONTALIS

TEMPORALIS

CORRUGATOR

PROCERUS

ORBICULARIS
OCULI

LEVATOR
PALPEBRAE

NASALIS

QUADRATUS LABII
SUPERIORIS

ZYGOMATICUS MINOR

BUCCINATOR

ZYGOMATICUS MAJOR

MASSETER

QUADRATUS LABII INFERIORIS

MENTALIS

ORBICULARIS
ORIS

PLATYSMA

INTERNAL MUSCLES OF THE JAW
(SIDE VIEW)

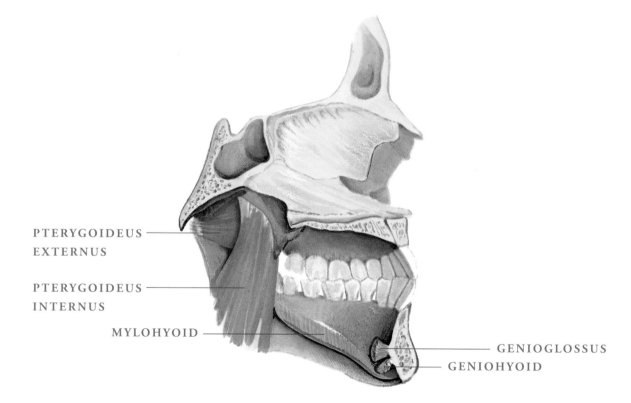

PTERYGOIDEUS
EXTERNUS

PTERYGOIDEUS
INTERNUS

MYLOHYOID

GENIOGLOSSUS
GENIOHYOID

MUSCLES OF THE HEAD, FACE, AND NECK
(SIDE VIEW)

GALEA APONEUROTICA

FRONTALIS

ORBICULARIS OCULI

PROCERUS

TEMPORALIS

DILATATOR NARIS
POSTERIOR

OCCIPITALIS

DILATATOR NARIS
ANTERIOR

NASALIS

DEPRESSOR
SEPTI

ORBICULARIS ORIS

STERNOCLEIDOMASTOID

TRAPEZIUS

MENTALIS

CANINUS

BUCCINATOR

PLATYSMA

MASSETER

PART TWO

CHAPTER 4

THE EXERCISES

WHEN YOU FIRST BEGIN the Facial Fitness

program, I recommend that you perform the exercises

and massage techniques in front of a mirror to ensure proper

hand placement, and to make sure that you are doing them

correctly. It is also advisable for you to begin by doing

them in the morning or in the evening when your face is

freshly cleansed and you are in a relaxed state. Try to dedicate

at least fifteen minutes to your facial exercise program at first,

and soon you will become so familiar with the techniques

that you will be able to perform them anywhere, anytime.

You may find that you are holding your breath while doing the exercises. That is fine for the ten-second duration of each exercise, but make sure to take a deep, cleansing breath when you complete the exercise, and remember to breathe normally between each set.

Before you begin, make sure your hands are thoroughly washed and, if possible, apply moisturizer to your face to help prevent unnecessary stretching of the facial skin.

The Facial Fitness program consists of twelve basic exercises designed to work many of the fifty-seven muscles of the face and neck synergistically, creating a stronger and more toned appearance. Once you have achieved the initial benefits of the Facial Fitness program, you will be ready to move on to the more advanced techniques to fur-ther sculpt and enhance your youthful look.

These techniques can be added to your daily facial exercise routine gradually, and you may increase the hold duration and number of repetitions to advance your workout even further. You should feel the muscles begin to fatigue, or "burn." This is a good sign. It means you are working effec-tively. (If you are using these exercises for rehabilitative purposes, however, you should stop before you feel the muscle fatigue.) Remember to relax and breathe normally between each set.

When you finish the Facial Fitness routine, you should feel completely relaxed and your skin will look rested and rejuve-nated immediately. Repeat these facial exer-cises once a day for the first three weeks, then every other day to maintain your toned and youthful appearance.

THE BASIC EXERCISES

THE ADVANCED EXERCISES

THE FOREHEAD LIFT

This exercise works the *galea aponeurotica*, *frontalis*, and *corrugator*
muscles to help diminish horizontal lines on the forehead.

Place the index fingers flat along the hairline.
While pushing up with the index fingers, push down
with the eyebrows. Hold down for 10 seconds.
Repeat 3 times, each time to the count of 10.

THE NASAL-LABIAL LINE DIMINISHER

This exercise works the muscles surrounding the nose
and mouth called the *orbicularis oris* and the *caninus,* and is designed
to help diminish the lines on either side of the mouth, referred to
as the nasal-labial lines, or marionette lines.

Open your mouth wide, making your face very long.
With your mouth open, slowly say, "ooh, ooh, ooh, ooh"
10 times. By vocalizing this sound, you will make the muscles
surrounding the mouth contract and relax, thereby
strengthening the surrounding muscles.

FACIAL FITNESS

THE NOSE THINNER

Did you know that your nose and ears continue to grow throughout your life because of the cartilage they contain? After all, W.C. Fields wasn't born with that nose. This exercise will strengthen the muscles that run across and alongside the nose, called the *nasalis,* the *procerus,* and the *depressor septi,* and will help keep your nose looking long and slim.

Push the tip of the nose down and flare your nostrils for 10 seconds. Repeat 3 times, each time to the count of 10.

This exercise is recommended for the treatment of Bell's palsy.

THE MOUTH LIFTER

This exercise will tone and train the muscles near the corners
of the mouth to lift, creating a more youthful appearance. The muscles affected
are the *orbicularis oris,* the *quadratus labii superioris,* the *quadratus
labii inferioris,* and the *caninus.*

Tighten the corners of your mouth very hard
and pull your lips together. Hold for 10 seconds.
Repeat 3 times, each time to the count of 10.

This exercise is recommended for the treatment of Bell's palsy.

THE LIP PUMPER

This exercise will help increase blood flow to the lips
and the surrounding muscles, known as the *orbicularis oris* and
the *mentalis,* to create a more full and pouty appearance.

Hold your mouth in a hard pout and try to smile.
While holding this position, try to force a small stream
of air out, just at the center of the lips. Hold your
finger in the front of the lips to ensure that the air stream
is thin and steady. Hold for 10 seconds and then relax
and breathe normally. Repeat 3 times,
each time to the count of 10.

This exercise is recommended for the treatment of Bell's palsy.

THE NECK STRENGTHENER

This exercise strengthens the muscles in both the front and back of your neck, known as the *platysma,* the *sternocleidomastoid,* and the *trapezius* muscles. This exercise may also be done while lying down on your back.

Move your head forward, leading with your bottom jaw. Extend your neck as far forward as you can and hold that position for 10 seconds. Then return to the original position. Repeat this exercise 3 times, holding each extension for 10 seconds.

FACIAL FITNESS

THE JAWLINE ENHANCER

This exercise works the muscles surrounding the jaw—
called the *masseter,* the *pterygoideus internus* and *externus,* the *temporalis,*
and the *buccinator*—as well as the muscles under the chin, such as
the *platysma,* helping to tone and tighten this delicate area.

Place your hand palm side down under your chin.
While holding your hand steady for resistance,
push your chin down against your hand 10 times.
Do 3 sets of 10 and then relax.

THE NECK AND JAWLINE TONER

This technique tones and tightens the *platysma* muscles,
located at the front of the neck as well as on the sides. It also
helps tone the muscles that support the jawline.

Tilt your head back, extending your bottom jaw.
Feel that the neck is tightened up and hold for 10 seconds.
Repeat 3 times, each time to the count of 10.

This exercise is recommended for the treatment of TMJ disorder.

THE NECK AND JAWLINE ENHANCER

Again, this technique is designed to tone the *platsyma* muscle
and other muscles along the jawline, helping to prevent
a double chin as well as the appearance of jowls.

Turn your head to the right, extend your jaw
and hold for 10 seconds. Return your head back to center.
Now turn your head to the left, extend your jaw,
and hold for 10 seconds. Repeat this exercise 3 times
on each side, each time to the count of 10.

THE VERTICAL LINE DIMINISHER

This exercise is designed to flatten and relax the muscles that
you use when you frown, such as the *frontalis* and the *procerus* muscles,
and to minimize the appearance of deep vertical lines.

Gently grasp the skin on either side of your face,
just above your nose and between your eyebrows where vertical
lines tend to form. Pull gently in an outward direction
while pushing down with the inside corners of the eyebrows.
Hold for 10 seconds. Repeat 3 times, each time
to the count of 10.

THE TOP EYELID LIFTER

Similar in technique to the Forehead Lift, this exercise is designed to strengthen the upper eyelid muscle, known as the *levator palpebrae,* by opening up the eye and lifting the brow.

Place your index fingers flat under the eyebrows. Gently push up with your fingers while pushing down with both eyebrows. Hold to the count of 10. Repeat 3 times, each time to the count of 10.

THE UNDER-EYE LINE DIMINISHER

Designed to strengthen the muscles below and around the eyes, known as the *orbicularis oculi,* this technique is essential to reducing puffiness, and it also diminishes the lines that form around the delicate eye area.

Gently place your middle and ring fingers at the outside corners of your eyes. Squinting with the lower eye muscles, squeeze and release 10 times. Repeat this exercise 3 times, squeezing and releasing 10 times each.

FACIAL FITNESS

ADVANCED JAWLINE TONERS

These techniques further strengthen the *platsyma* muscle under
the chin and along the jawline, as well as the *masseter*.

EXERCISE #1

Depress your tongue firmly against the roof of your
mouth, tilt your head back slightly, and hold this position
for 10 seconds. Repeat 3 times, each time to the count of 10.

This exercise is recommended for the treatment of TMJ disorder.

EXERCISE #2

Pull your cheeks back towards your ears (using only your
facial muscles). Feel the ears lift and hold this position
for 10 seconds. Repeat 3 times, each time to the count of 10.

THE NOSE DEFINER

This technique will define the nose even more by strengthening the *nasalis* and *depressor septi*.

Hold the tip of your nose slightly with your thumb and index finger. Don't squeeze too hard, you want to be able to feel the nostrils flare 10 times and relax. Do 3 sets, flaring your nostrils 10 times for each set.

THE UPPER LIP
LINE ERASER

By further toning the *mentalis* muscle, the vertical lines
on the upper lip will begin to diminish.

Press your index finger against the cleft
between the lip and nose. Smile with your mouth
slightly ajar and hold for 10 seconds.
Repeat 3 times, each time to the count of 10.

HEAD LIFTS FOR DOUBLE CHIN

This exercise helps increase the strength
and stability of both the front and the back of the neck
and tightens the *platsyma* muscles.

Lie down on your back on the floor.
Lift your head straight up, leading with your chin.
Hold for 3 seconds, then relax. Repeat this 10 times
and relax. You may do as many as 3 sets of 10,
but work up to this gradually to avoid neck strain.

FACIAL FITNESS

THE EYE TONER

This technique is designed to further strengthen
the *orbicularis oculi,* and to diminish the appearance of fine lines
and wrinkles around the eyes.

Pull the innermost corners of your eyes up
and hold for 2 seconds. Repeat 10 times and relax.
You may do as many as 3 sets of 10 repetitions.

CHAPTER 5

THE MASSAGE TECHNIQUES

M ASSAGE has been practiced for centuries and is considered among the oldest forms of healing. With regular facial massage you can have firmer, smoother skin by increasing the skin's temperature, which causes the skin to release toxins and impurities that cleansers alone cannot reach. Beneath the skin's surface, massage enhances the action of the lymphatic system by moving bacteria and waste away from the skin cells so these toxins can be eliminated. Facial massage also strengthens and tones the facial muscles, and prevents wrinkling and sagging. Massage of the face and neck increases circulation by maximizing cellular turnover and brings nutrients to the skin's surface to give you a more radiant appearance. It is also very effective in helping to relieve stress. When you feel stressed, the muscles in your face contract. This often results in headaches, jaw pain, and even neck pain, and can cause deep wrinkling. Massage relaxes the muscles, releases tension, and helps to revive the spirit.

The Facial Fitness massage techniques were designed to complement the Facial Fitness exercises. You may perform these techniques after you exercise your face, however it is recommended that you create a calm, serene environment in which to do the massages. Perhaps you can light a scented candle and play some soft music in the room where you're doing your massages. Before you begin the massage techniques, remember to thoroughly cleanse your face and neck and apply your facial moisturizing cream to both. Besides helping the fingers glide over the skin and ensuring smooth, even strokes, applying moisturizer minimizes the risk of stretching your skin. Make sure to reapply the moisturizing cream as needed. Work with gentle, rhythmic strokes, matching the movements to your breathing.

Like the exercises, you should do these techniques once a day for the first three weeks, and then you can downgrade to once every other day.

THE MASSAGE TECHNIQUES

THE NECK SWEEP

This massage will increase circulation to the neck
and eliminate any puffiness.

While applying moisturizer with your fingertips,
sweep in an upward and outward direction, beginning
at the collarbone and going up your neck with
your hands turned slightly outward. Cover the entire neck
while turning your head from side to side 5 times.

THE MASSAGE TECHNIQUES

THE ADVANCED NECK MASSAGE

Like the Neck Sweep, this massage is designed to increase circulation and help rid the area of any fluid buildup.

With hands open and palms facing down, using the backs of your fingers, roll your hands forward under your chin, each hand following the other for 10 seconds. Repeat as needed.

THE SKIN GRASP

This technique will help to rejuvenate the elasticity
of the facial skin.

Gently grasp the skin just above the jawline
with your thumbs, index fingers, and middle fingers.
Slowly, pushing up with the thumbs, grasp the skin,
creeping up toward the eye. Begin again at the
jawline, rolling up toward the ear. Around the forehead,
walk fingers up around the hairline. Begin again
at the inside corners of the eyebrows, rolling outward
to each temple. Repeat as needed.

THE BETWEEN-BROW MASSAGE

This area of the face is the most prone to developing deep vertical lines.
This technique helps to relax this area instantly.

With the tips of your fingers, gently massage
the area between your eyebrows 25 times in a small
circular motion. Repeat again in the other direction.
Apply more moisturizer, if necessary.

THE EYE AND BROW MASSAGE

This stimulating technique increases circulation and helps
to flush out built-up fluid around the eyes.

Apply eye cream with your ring fingers
(because they provide the lightest touch) to the eye area
in a gentle, tapping motion. Then, in a circular motion,
gently massage the area around the eye from the
inside to the outside, around and around, 10 times.
Finish by gently tapping under the eye to promote
circulation and reduce puffiness.

THE FOREHEAD MASSAGE

**Much like the massage for the eyes, this will help to eliminate
any fluid buildup and relax the *frontalis* muscle.**

With your fingertips, gently massage your skin,
making a semicircle on the forehead above the eyebrows.
Expand the motion outward toward the temple areas and back.
Finish by massaging the temple areas in a circular motion,
then stop and apply slight pressure to the temples for
a moment, and release. Repeat as needed.

THE SCALP LIFT

This relaxing method of massage increases circulation to the scalp, which will promote hair growth as well as relieve tension.

Place both hands under your hair on the scalp. Gently lift the hair from the roots and hold for 3 seconds. Repeat this technique all over the scalp, making sure to cover the entire head.

THE FROWN RELIEVER

This technique is designed to relax the muscles that
cause vertical frown lines to form.

Place your index and middle fingers just inside
the eyebrows. While applying slight pressure to the area,
gently sweep upward toward the center of the forehead
and hold for a moment while applying slight pressure
for 3 seconds. Repeat as needed.

This massage is recommended for the treatment of Bell's palsy.

THE CHEEKBONE RELAXER

This massage increases facial circulation and
also helps clear the sinuses.

Starting at the corners of the nose, apply slight
pressure to the nose with your index finger. Sweep
out toward the ears and hold for 3 seconds.
Repeat as needed.

EAR TENSION RELEASE

This technique is great for relieving tension all over.

Starting at the earlobes, squeeze to apply slight
pressure and hold for 3 seconds. Sliding upward toward
the back of the ear, again apply slight pressure
and hold for 3 seconds. Finish at the top of the ear.
Repeat the cycle 3 times.

You may also pull backward gently on the ear
for more relief when you are finished.

THE FACE PRESS

This massage increases circulation, eliminates puffiness,
and relaxes the muscles of the face and neck.

Sit down and rest your elbows on your lap.
Turn your palms up and rest your forehead on the palms
of your hands. Fully support the weight of your head
in your hands and relax your neck completely. Breathe
deeply and relax. Hold for 5 seconds.

Moving down to the eye area, place your
closed eyes in the palms of your hands and relax
completely. Hold for 5 seconds.

Now, move over to the cheeks and hold for 5 seconds.

Next, move down to the chin and jawline and again
hold for 5 seconds.

Finally, turn your hands outward and finish
with the front and sides of your neck, making sure
not to stretch the skin. When you are finished
sit up, breathe normally, and relax.

PART THREE

CHAPTER 6

HEALTHY LIFESTYLE, HEALTHY SKIN

I T'S NO SECRET that lifestyle choices greatly affect the way you look and feel. Your lifestyle has a critical impact on how your face and body show signs of aging. By making smart choices, you can significantly reduce the rate at which your skin begins to show these outward signs. By doing the Facial Fitness exercises and massage techniques, eating right, protecting your skin from the elements, and choosing beneficial skin-care products, you can stay looking fabulous well into your forties, fifties, sixties, and beyond.

As you may know, the skin is the largest organ in the body. It must have proper care and nutrition to carry out its vital functions. Primarily, the skin protects the internal systems of the body and acts as a barrier against the outer elements. It also helps keep you hydrated and regulates your body temperature through the sweat glands. It allows you to feel sensations like pain and warns you of potential harm. It's also a good indicator of internal health. For example, if your skin begins to turn yellowish, it may be an indication of serious illness, such as jaundice or liver cancer. So make sure you take care of your skin, because you only have one!

CLEANSERS, MOISTURIZERS, AND COSMETICS

Of course, you need to be as concerned about what goes onto your skin as you are about what goes into your body. Every substance that comes in contact with your skin that can be absorbed—and most can—reaches your internal organs in about twenty-six seconds. It is not just for the sake of your skin that you wash off potentially hazardous materials and liquids as soon as possible. It is because they are being absorbed deep within your body almost instantly.

Now think about what is in your cosmetics and skin-care products. Don't really know? Well, you had better start reading those labels more carefully. Many large cosmetics companies use synthetic or petrochemical ingredients in their skin-care products. Mineral oil, a by-product of the distillation of gasoline from crude oil, is one such ingredient, and is commonly used in lotions and baby oil.

Mineral oil and other petroleum-derived ingredients form a seal on the skin that traps moisture in but clogs the pores and prevents the skin from breathing and eliminating toxins. Mineral oil can also be harmful if ingested or inhaled, making it an especially hazardous choice for use on babies. Because of these dangers, the medical community has condemned the use of mineral oil taken orally or as an ingredient in medications. However, it is still available in many cosmetics and personal-care products, so let the buyer beware.

Cosmetics and personal-care products containing animal products or by-products should also be avoided. Remains from slaughterhouses and other places where dead animals are collected after being killed are combined in one big vat and boiled down in what are called rendering plants.

The fat and other substances are removed and then sold to large cosmetics companies. These then become key ingredients in the manufacturing of many products, such as lipsticks. I don't know about you, but I'm not putting that on my skin. I only recommend and use skin-care products that consist of natural, plant-based ingredients and other essential nutrients. They may cost a bit more, but for me—and for you—they are well worth it.

Some cosmetic and skin-care products contain carcinogenic or otherwise toxic ingredients that can damage your skin or be detrimental to your overall health. To learn more, I suggest reading a fascinating book by Christine H. Farlow, D.C., called *Dying To Look Good*. According to the book, some of the ingredients you should be aware of and avoid are:

- **Fragrances:** Each has up to six hundred different ingredients that may not be listed on the label.

- **Preservatives:** These may contain formaldehyde, which is a carcinogen, neurotoxin, irritant, and sensitizer.

- **Talc:** This is a known carcinogen and is not recommended for use on children.

- **Artificial colors:** Many of these cause cancer. D&C and FD&C colors are derived from coal tar, a known cancer-causing agent.

- **Silica:** While it is not harmful by itself, it may be contaminated with crystalline silica, which causes cancer.

- **Propylene glycol and sodium lauryl sulfate:** Common ingredients in shampoos, these are both skin irritants. If ingested, propylene glycol can cause kidney and liver damage, and sodium laurel sulfate degenerates cell membranes and can alter the genetic information in cells, as well as damage the immune system.

Dying to Look Good is a great reference that will help you identify hundreds of dangerous ingredients in well-known brands and guide you toward selecting safer products. Be smart and keep yourself informed by researching and finding the best products available to make you look your best, and steer clear of those with questionable ingredients. Here's a good rule to follow: if you can't pronounce it, you may want to avoid it.

Now that you know some of the ingredients your cosmetic and skin-care products should not contain, here are a few of the beneficial ingredients that they should contain.

Look for products containing retinol, or vitamin A, which is essential for the maintenance of your skin, as well as for your overall health. Vitamin A may be incorporated into both prescription and over-the-counter products and is very effective in rejuvenating skin cells. Skin treated with vitamin A will appear smoother and have a better texture and fewer dark spots (also known as age spots). The sooner you start using a retinoid, the better. The results will be dramatic.

DMAE, or dimenthylaminoethanol, is a phenomenal ingredient that helps protect skin cells and acts as an antioxidant, preventing damage from free radicals. Free radicals are atoms with an uneven number of electrons in their outer shell. This means that one electron is unpaired, making it chemically reactive, so the atom will now try to steal an electron from a neighboring molecule to stabilize itself. By stealing molecules from others, they in turn create more free radicals in the process. They damage healthy cells, especially those of collagen. The damaged collagen becomes stiff and is no longer flexible, so the skin begins to look old or damaged.

Another beneficial ingredient is copper peptide, which helps heal the skin. EGF, or epidermal growth factor, is another amazing substance. This protein promotes skin-cell growth, creating firmer skin with regular use. Coenzyme Q10, another vitamin, is an antioxidant that also fights free radical damage in the skin cells. Alpha-lipoic acid is a fatty acid that fights free radicals and helps protect the skin. One of the most popular ingredients in skin-care today is vitamin C. However, make sure you look for products that say "stabilized vitamin C" on the label, or better yet, those containing vitamin C ester. Another fabulous ingredient that has been proven to fight inflammation, free radical damage, and irritation, as well as promote healing, is vitamin E, or tocotrienol.

All of these substances have been shown to be very beneficial to your skin. Each of these ingredients works in its own miraculous way to improve the skin's health, tone, and texture.

Products made from natural plant extracts or plant-based ingredients, without harsh soaps or chemicals, are better for your overall health and provide a greater benefit for the skin. They are readily available in the marketplace and are suitable for most skin types. But beware, just because it says

"botanical" does not necessarily mean it is safe for all people to use. Some of the most toxic and allergenic substances in the world are derived from plants, so it is important to know what you are allergic to before you choose a new skin-care line. Read the label of every product carefully if you have any known allergies and test a small amount on a less conspicuous area than the face to make sure you are not allergic to it.

That said, many botanical ingredients have been proven safe and effective in helping to improve the skin's quality. Some botanical ingredients, such as green tea, aloe vera, ginkgo biloba, and echinacea have been shown to reduce inflammation in the skin. Green tea contains powerful antioxidants. When taken orally, these antioxidants act as a natural combatant that contributes to healthy cells by absorbing harmful free radicals. When applied topically, such as in a cream, it does the same for the skin. Aloe vera, a plant that has been used for centuries to heal wounds, has been shown to improve overall healing and relieve skin irritations.

⊱ ⊰ ⊱

Products made from natural plant extracts or plant-based ingredients, without harsh soaps or chemicals, are better for your overall health and provide a greater benefit for the skin.

⊱ ⊰ ⊱

Skin-care products containing both vitamins and botanicals have been proven to enhance overall health and the appearance of the skin. Over time, they can even undo some of the environmental damage we suffer from toxins in the air and water by promoting healing and offering protection from environmental toxins.

As mentioned previously, it is also important to include a broad-spectrum sunscreen in your daily skin-care routine by either choosing a day cream with an SPF of fifteen or higher, or using sunscreen alone before you apply your other skin care products. The greatest skin-care products in the world won't make a difference if you continue to accelerate the aging process by failing to protect your skin from exposure to the sun. I cannot stress this point enough: don't leave home without sunscreen.

Your basic skin-care routine should consist of cleansing, toning, and moisturizing. Remember to read labels so you can avoid products that contain harsh soaps or fragrances, and choose products that are formulated for your particular skin type, be it normal, oily, dry, or a combination of these. Use a gentle skin cleanser and try to cleanse your face twice a day. If you can only cleanse once a day, do it at night, before you go to bed.

Sleeping with makeup on your face is one sure way to get acne and dull skin. Consult with a dermatologist if you have a condition that may increase your skin's sensitivity, such as eczema, psoriasis, or acne. A gentle exfoliator used occasionally will help the skin look more radiant by removing dead skin cells. But it can also remove some of the protective cells from the skin's surface, so don't overdo it.

GOOD NUTRITION

As mentioned earlier, the skin looks its best when properly hydrated from within. Moisturizing is great, but most creams just draw water from within the skin's layers and hold it on top for a while. Drinking plenty of water, preferably distilled, will keep your skin looking great and your body functioning properly, because water provides a good infusion of oxygen to all areas of the body. Why is distilled water better? It is thought that distilled water is neutrally charged, or has no charge. Therefore, as it passes through your system it picks up those harmful free radicals and flushes them out more effectively than non-distilled water.

A few vitamin lines available today are specially formulated with high levels of antioxidants. These vitamins come in both pill and liquid form and have been proven to help protect and repair the skin from within. Look for formulations containing green tea, grapeseed, and beta carotene, and add these to your daily routine.

❧ ❧ ❧

Not only does proper nutrition oxygenate the cells, but it provides the antioxidants needed to fight off attacks from free radicals that bombard you.

❧ ❧ ❧

I cannot stress enough how important good nutrition is to the skin. By consuming the vital nutrients and vitamins needed for the body to thrive and repair itself, you are helping the skin cells regenerate faster. Not only does proper nutrition oxygenate the cells, but it provides the antioxidants needed to fight off attacks from free radicals that bombard you on a continual basis. A well-balanced diet, designed to bolster your overall health as well as the skin's appearance, includes oily fishes such as tuna, mackerel, and salmon, which are filled with beneficial omega-3 fatty acids and are excellent sources of protein. Skinless chicken, turkey, eggs, yogurt, and cheese are also excellent sources of protein. And let's not forget veggies. Green, leafy vegetables such as escarole, spinach, and arugula are all excellent sources of vitamins and nutrients. Avocado, asparagus, cauliflower, broccoli, and eggplant are bursting with vitamins, minerals, and antioxidants as well. Garlic has many health benefits, as do tomatoes and peppers.

Some fruits to add to your diet are strawberries, cherries, kiwis, and blackberries. Choosing organic produce is always best. If organic produce is not readily available in your area, make sure you wash your fruits and vegetables thoroughly before eating or cooking, since many of them are treated with pesticides. Some fruits, such as strawberries, hold on to what they are treated with more than others, so be sure to wash them more than once. You should also consume strawberries shortly after you remove the green leafy stem, because once the skin is cut, the strawberry begins to lose its vitamin potency.

Some healthy snack alternatives are naturally dried fruits, nuts, olives, and raw vegetables. Of course, before you start adding any of these foods to your diet, make sure you are not allergic to them or intolerant of them. Another tip for good eating habits is to try to prepare foods with olive oil, as opposed to other types of oils or margarine, because it contains more nutri-

ents. Always smell the oil before you use it; oil may become rancid, and rancid oil has a toxic effect on the body.

Try to cut down on the amount of sugar you eat. Besides promoting tooth decay and adding empty calories to your diet, sugar can also make acne worse. Chocolate, while not completely hazardous because of the benefits from the flavonoids it contains, should be kept to a minimum as well. Limit the amount of salt you use to flavor the foods you eat and avoid seasoned salts that contain MSG, because it may cause headaches.

Use butter or spreadable margarine (the kind that comes in a tub) in moderation, but avoid margarine and shortening that comes in stick form. These products undergo hydrogenation to turn them from a liquid to a solid, and to extend their shelf life. Hydrogenated oils—which are also found in fried foods, fast foods, pastries, cookies, and other snacks—contain high levels of trans fatty acids, which raise LDL ("bad") cholesterol levels and lower HDL ("good") cholesterol levels, and increase the risk of developing heart disease and stroke.

❦ ❦ ❦

Try to chew food on both sides of your mouth to prevent alignment problems with your jaw and teeth, and to maintain normal function.

❦ ❦ ❦

It may seem like an odd thing to be aware of, but for those who want to avoid any potential problems with TMJ disorder, or for anyone currently suffering from it,

you should try to be aware of which side of your mouth you are chewing your food on. Try to chew food on both sides of your mouth to prevent alignment problems with your jaw and teeth, and to maintain normal function. If you usually eat on the right side, try eating on the left side once in a while.

As you are probably aware, cigarette smoking is by far one of the worst habits you can develop. Smokers will tell you that smoking can quickly become an addiction that's not easily overcome. Besides the proven correlation between smoking and various cancers, emphysema, and other serious illnesses and diseases, smoking is one of the biggest causes of premature aging. The carcinogenic chemicals contained in cigarettes reduce the skin's elasticity. Smoking also creates an abundance of unchallenged free radicals, which accelerate the aging process, not to mention all the squinting and puckering going on whenever one drags on a cigarette. Just look at the mouth of someone who smokes. The vertical lines surrounding their mouth are a telltale sign of years spent smoking.

PHYSICAL AND EMOTIONAL HEALTH

Aside from the products you put directly on your body or into your body, a number of other factors affect the way your skin looks. The position in which you sleep can greatly affect the way you look in the morning. Sleeping facedown with your face buried in a pillow will certainly guarantee a puffy, line-filled complexion. And sleeping on one side or the other will crease the face and cause lines that over time will become permanent.

Try to sleep on your back with your head slightly elevated on a pillow to reduce swelling or creasing on your face. If you must sleep on your side, position the pillow behind your ear and away from your face so that you are not creasing your face and causing permanent sleep lines.

Getting enough rest is one of the most important ways to help your body regenerate and heal, so make sure to get at least eight hours of sleep each night. Taking an occasional afternoon nap is also great. Getting just a few minutes of extra sleep in the afternoon will rejuvenate and recharge your batteries before you head off for a busy evening.

"Never underestimate the power of laughter." Whoever said that first couldn't have been more correct. With all that you endure in a day, and all the challenges you face from moment to moment, it's a wonder how you manage to keep your sense of humor. But smile you must. First of all, smiling is good for your facial muscles. And don't worry if it causes lines around your eyes, just do your eye exercises and you'll look great. As practitioners of mind-body health have known for centuries, being happy is vital to good health. So try to surround yourself with happy, positive people and good friends as much as you can.

As practitioners of mind-body health have known for centuries, being happy is vital to good health.

Laughing out loud with my friends, playing with my children, drinking great red wine, riding my horses, and being in love are all things that make me happy. Your idea of happiness may be entirely different, but remember that your personal happiness is the goal, so try to make time to do what you enjoy as often as you can.

Taking a walk daily can do wonders for the body as well as the soul. Take a few deep breaths and remember to swing your arms rhythmically to reeducate and balance the brain. It is great exercise and the endorphin release makes you feel fantastic.

Allow yourself to live life to the fullest and enjoy every minute by living in the present. Don't worry about mistakes you've made in the past or what may lie ahead in the future. Living in the present will make such a difference in how you look and feel, and it will make you much more attractive to those around you.

QUICK FIXES FOR THE FACE AND HAIR

So you just woke up and your face is puffy and tired-looking. It happens to everyone. Maybe you partied a little too much or you just couldn't fall asleep. Whatever the reason, there are a few things you can do to remedy this. First, start by taking a nice warm shower and thoroughly cleansing and exfoliating your face. Finish your cleansing routine by running cool water over your face and gently pat dry. Apply your toner and let it air-dry.

ஜ ஜ ஜ

Apply your makeup sparingly, as it tends to settle into fine lines, making you look older.

ஜ ஜ ஜ

When washing and especially drying your face, avoid rubbing the skin too hard. Try not to stretch the skin with your hands by rubbing your eyes when you're tired. As a matter of fact, try to avoid touching your face during the day as much as possible, because as you know, your hands are not always clean and the dirt and bacteria can cause breakouts.

After washing your face and applying your toner, apply your eye cream with your ring finger in a gentle tapping motion all around the eye area. Let each product dry for a few moments before applying the next one. Now, apply your moisturizer (one that contains one or more of the recommended ingredients) to your face and neck and do each of your Facial Fitness exercises. Follow that by doing all of the Facial Fitness massage techniques, except the scalp lift (we'll save that for later). This will help eliminate any fluid buildup that causes puffiness, especially around the eyes, and increase circulation to eliminate any toxin buildup. If your moisturizer does not contain sunscreen, apply some now. Apply your makeup sparingly, as it tends to settle into fine lines, making you look older.

If you wake up with a new addition to your complexion in the form of a mini–Mount St. Helens, here are a few tips that can quickly remedy the problem. When your skin breaks out, you should never squeeze the blemish before it is ready. This can cause swelling and terrible scarring. After thoroughly cleansing your face, you should apply heat, such as a warm compress, to bring the pimple to a head, and then apply a topical medication or clay mask to dry it out. You can also try apply-

ing ice to the pimple to reduce the redness and swelling. Ice causes blood vessels to shrink temporarily. Another good remedy to try is to crush an aspirin and add a drop of water to it to form a paste. Apply this aspirin paste directly to the pimple. Aspirin contains salicylic acid, which is the same ingredient found in acne-control products. Do not use this aspirin paste if you are allergic to aspirin.

Regular visits to the dermatologist can help keep acne under control and minimize the occurrence of breakouts. Your dermatologist can prescribe medications and treatments designed to prevent breakouts from occurring in the first place. I am a great fan of facials and find them to be beneficial for many reasons. First of all, they are a relaxing indulgence that I think everyone should experience. Secondly, they remove dirt, makeup, and built-up oils trapped deep within the skin and leave the face really clean. Finally, the rejuvenating facial massage is wonderful for the circulation and helps to release toxins built up within the skin's layers. Try to either get a professional facial at least once a month, or give yourself a facial at home. The extra care you lavish on your skin will show in both the skin's tone and its radiance. Just make sure you use quality products that contain pure ingredients. Many salons and spas have excellent products available for purchase so that you can achieve similar results at home.

To help get back that healthy look from within, start by drinking two or three glasses of water and a cup of green tea, if you have it. If you don't, it's time to go get some and add it to your daily routine. The antioxidants contained in green tea help rid the body of toxins, absorb free radicals, and decrease inflammation in the skin. Take a vitamin high in antioxidants and make sure to eat a breakfast rich in protein and nutrients, such as egg whites, oatmeal, melon, and some fresh tomatoes. These tips will have you looking and feeling better in no time.

❧ ❧ ❧

Try to either get a professional facial at least once a month, or give yourself a facial at home.

❧ ❧ ❧

So what about that hair? Has it lost its luster and shine? Well, here are a few tips to help increase circulation to the scalp and bring back some of the shine that can be stripped away by overuse of hair-care products. While in the shower, shampoo your hair twice. Use a shampoo that is right for your particular type of hair, like a deep moisturizing formula if your hair is dry and brittle. It is a good idea to use a clarifying shampoo once a week to remove built-up residue on the hair left by styling products. Follow by applying a moisturizing pack containing protein and let it sit on your hair for a few minutes while you begin your skin-care regimen. Keep a wide-toothed comb in the shower and comb the conditioner through your hair before you rinse it out. Rinse your hair with cool water, with your head tilted back, to keep as much of the conditioner as possible off your freshly cleansed face. Wrap your wet hair gently with a soft towel. Apply a leave-in conditioner with detangler to your hair and comb it through to the ends. Style hair as usual, but before you apply any type of finishing product to the hair, such as hairspray, perform the scalp lift massage technique to increase circulation and relieve stress.

If you don't already own a bonnet dryer, consider investing in one. Once a week, apply a protein pack to your hair, or if you don't have one on hand, put olive oil into a spray bottle and spray your hair until it's saturated, cover with a plastic shower cap, and sit under the dryer for fifteen minutes. Thoroughly wash out the oil, and your hair will look and feel incredibly soft and shiny. Most beauty supply stores carry bonnet dryers and protein pack conditioners.

COSMETIC OPTIONS AND FACIAL FITNESS

The question has arisen on numerous occasions whether or not you can start exercising your face once you have had a cosmetic procedure, such as collagen or restylane injections. The answer is a resounding yes. According to the American Society of Aesthetic Plastic Surgery, cosmetic procedures consisting of filler injectables such as restylane have increased over 650 percent from 2003 to 2004. The latest data on 2005 is not yet available, but it would be safe to say that it will be an even higher percentage, based on the increased popularity and availability of these procedures. Because these injectable fillers do not cause partial paralysis in the facial muscles, as does Botox, the muscles can still be toned and strengthened effectively as an adjunct to these procedures.

Botox, or botulinum toxin type A, is a purified derivative of botulism. The puri-fied toxin is diluted and directly injected into the facial muscles, restricting the ability to contract that particular muscle. Used primarily on the frontalis muscle and around the outermost part of the eye muscles, this temporary effect makes it somewhat difficult to effectively exercise these muscles. If you are doing facial exercises and want to continue to do so for the remaining muscles of the face and neck, by all means you may do so without worry of undoing the effects of the Botox. Incidentally, immediately after the Botox injection has been administered, it is recommended that the patient do facial exercises for at least two hours to help the Botox work more effectively.

This is not exactly what the Facial Fitness program was designed for, but if you do choose to go the Botox route, well then, there is one more way to use the facial exercises you have learned.

As mentioned earlier, plastic surgeons generally encourage the use of facial exercises both before and after facial cosmetic surgery as a way of enhancing and prolonging the effect of the procedure. So, if the surgical route is one you have already embarked on, or are considering embarking on, then you can make the Facial Fitness program part of your pre– and post– operative routine, if your physician advises you to do so.

CHAPTER 7

FINAL COMMENTS

THE TECHNIQUES AND TIPS I share with you in this book are designed to help you look and feel your best. By following a daily regimen of exercise, massage, good nutrition, and healthy lifestyle choices, you can reverse some of the visible signs of aging. With continued dedication to yourself, you will start to see the changes happen right before your eyes. People will begin to ask what you are doing differently and will want to know your secret. This proven method of toning and tightening the facial muscles will make you look years younger. And it only takes a few minutes a day.

❧ ❧ ❧

With continued dedication to yourself, you will start to see the changes happen right before your eyes.

❧ ❧ ❧

Good health and beauty start with a commitment to yourself, and a belief that you are worth it. To look and feel your best, you must make changes in your daily routine. For some, these are small changes, for others, this may mean changing everything. You should avoid habits and behaviors detrimental to your health and start making smart, well-informed choices. After all, it's never too late to make yourself a priority. Not only will the knowledge you gain be beneficial to your health, but to your children's health as well. You are your children's greatest teacher, so educate yourself about the potentially dangerous ingredients contained in many of the products that are on the market today and search for healthy alternatives. The Facial Fitness program was designed to be just that—a healthy alternative.

Incorporating all the essential components to healthy living into your daily regimen will guarantee that you look and feel your best, and it will show first and foremost on your face. You can achieve so many benefits from exercise and incorporating the Facial Fitness program into your daily routine, and this program will ensure that you keep your most visible asset looking great. It's never too late to start exercising your facial muscles. You are guaranteed to see results at any age.

❧ ❧ ❧

Consistency is the key, so don't give up if you don't see results immediately.

❧ ❧ ❧

As I mentioned earlier, because the muscles of the face are smaller than most, they respond to exercise rather quickly. Just remember to stick with it. Consistency is the key, so don't give up if you don't see results immediately. Remember: it took a lifetime to look the way you do now, so be patient and diligent, and soon you will begin to see an amazing transformation.

It has been my pleasure to share this information with you and I hope you will share it with others. Please refer back to this book and to the others I have recommended when you need inspiration, information, or simply to refresh your memory.

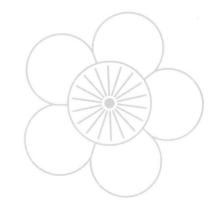

BIBLIOGRAPHY AND ADDITIONAL RESOURCES

The American Society for Aesthetic Plastic Surgery: http://www.surgery.org

Begoun, Paula. *The Beauty Bible.* Seattle: Beginning Press, 2002.

Bell's Palsy Research Foundation: http://www.bellspalsy.com

Colbert, Don, MD. *Toxic Relief.* Lake Mary, Florida: Siloam Press, 2003.

Farlow, D.C., Christine. *Dying To Look Good: The Disturbing Truth About What's Really In Your Cosmetics, Toiletries and Personal Care Products . . . And What You Can Do About It.* Escondido, CA: KISS For Health Publishing, 2006.

Herbal Luxuries, "Mineral Oil and Why You Should Avoid It," Herbal Luxuries, http://www.herballuxuries.com/mineral-oil.htm.

Lowe, Nicholas, MD. *Away With Wrinkles.* New York: Marlowe and Company, 2005.

Mohammed, Renea. "Animal Rendering Products In More Places Than You Think." *Animal Writes: The Vancouver Humane Society Newsletter.* Summer 2003.

Mitchell, Sandi, Ph.D. "Beauty, Pride and Pig Grease." *Health Freedom News.* Jan/Feb 1991.

The TMJ Association: http://www.tmj.org

INDEX